Energy ++

How To Supercharge Your Body
To
Get More Done

RON KNESS

Contents

Disclaimer

This publication is for informational purposes only and is not intended as medical advice. Medical advice should always be obtained from a qualified medical professional for any health conditions or symptoms associated with them.

Every possible effort has been made in preparing and researching this material. We make no warranties with respect to the accuracy, applicability of its contents or any omissions.

See your healthcare professional before starting any diet, health or exercise program!

Chapter 1: Why Energy Management > Time Management?

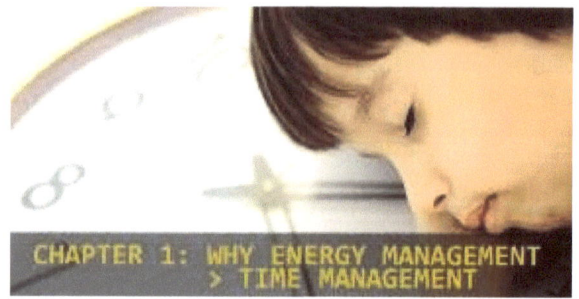

What is it that is holding you back in life? A lot of us make the mistaken assumption that it is time. We think that if only we had a little more time, then we could get all kinds of things done. If we had a little more time, then the house would be cleaner, we'd spend more time with our family and friends and we'd be able to progress faster through our career. Maybe we could start a new training program as well and finally get those abs?

But there just isn't time in the day. We work from 9-5 and when we get home, we often still have a long list of tasks to do that we just don't have time to finish. That includes checking the mail, paying bills, making dinner, washing up and hopefully getting just a little bit of time to spend with family!

Man, if only there were more time... right?

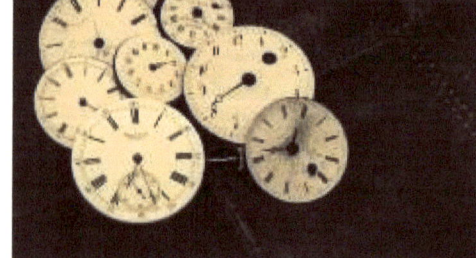

Well actually, time is very often *not* the problem. Rather, the problem comes down to energy.

Think about it: if you really don't have any time to do anything, then how were you able to watch that entire Boxset of *Game of Thrones* recently? If you really don't have time to do anything, then how have you been finding time to play *Uncharted*?

If you *genuinely* work and busy yourself from the first thing in the morning, all the way up until bedtime, then the answer would be simple: get up earlier, or go to bed later.

No, that is not the problem.

Instead, the problem is energy. Time management isn't the only big deal here: energy management is just as important. If you can't effectively manage your energy, then you're going to find that you can't make *full use* of your time. And that's a problem!

What probably *really* happens when you get home from work, is that you collapse onto the sofa and watch TV for a bit. Or maybe you just procrastinate a little by not really doing anything much for a short time.

Either way, you *could* be working. You *could* be working on that amazing novel.

The issue is not your time at all but rather it is your energy. And this isn't to say that you're in some way lazy, or that you *could* be making better use of your time right now. Instead, it is to say that you're simply pushing yourself too hard and too far – and it should come as no surprise that you're not achieving as much as you had hoped as a result.

Energy is something most of us ignore: 'I have a few hours tonight,' we say, 'I'll do it then!'. The only problem is that if you don't have the energy, then you're *not going to do it*.

Your energy, like time, is finite, it can only go so far, and if you ignore that fact then you're going to run out of steam and *not* accomplish the things you want to do.

Coming to Terms With Energy Management

There's a good chance that you may be reading this and considering energy management properly for the very first time. Perhaps it's something you never really thought about before – and you wouldn't be alone in that thinking!

But even at this early stage in the book, you've hopefully learned a valuable lesson. Simply acknowledging that energy (and not time) is probably what's holding you back is one of the very best things you can do to start making life easier.

Once you come to terms with this, you can start to think more logically and realistically about what you can achieve in a day. That means you can remove items from your agenda today to another day – knowing full well that you won't be able to accomplish them this day – and thus actually get *more* done as a result and come home with more energy left over to accomplish the things you want to do after work, but never had the energy to do before.

When thinking about whether you're going to walk home tonight or drive, be realistic and accept that driving *may* be easier. When planning to complete a long list of chores this evening, be honest with yourself and ask how likely you are to really complete that list; and do you really need to accomplish everything on that list tonight or can some things wait until tomorrow night? Did you manage to finish everything you set out to last time? Give yourself a break and organize your day sensibly.

Our Strategy for Boosting Energy

So what is our overall strategy for boosting energy?

It comes down to a few things. The first is management: managing our time better and thinking about how much energy we're likely to have in a given day and what we actually want to do with it. And by finding ways to avoid wasting energy, we can save more for the things that we ultimately decide really matter.

The next step is to start small and not be too ambitious. That's true with the other things we're trying to achieve and it's also true of the lifestyle changes we're introducing in this book. Simply put? You're not going to transform your energy levels and your health overnight – and you shouldn't try! Work up to it slowly and be smart about how you're raising your energy level. We're going to introduce the concept of 'kaizen' here, which means that we're introducing small changes with the aim of eventually seeing big results. Kaizen is a Japanese concept that basically means any journey is best accomplished with lots of little steps.

And finally, we're going to change *everything*. We're going to look at our health and our lifestyles holistically. We're going to acknowledge that to boost energy, it is not good enough that we simply introduce one new lifestyle habit, or start drinking smoothies. We need to rethink *everything*.

This book will be your guide and by the end the aim is for you to be *crackling* with energy. You should feel like a coiled spring ready to explode. And then you can achieve some truly amazing things!

Chapter Two: This Is Where Everything Changes

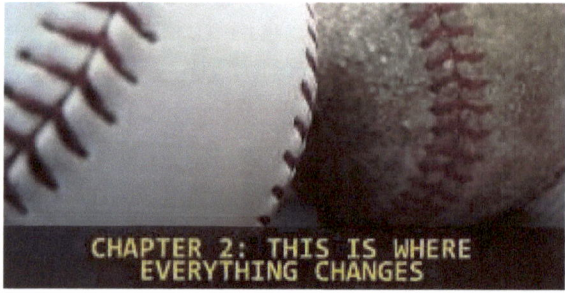

At the end of the last chapter, we mentioned that we had to change *everything*. That's a tall order but using the aforementioned 'kaizen' approach, we should see that it's relatively possible to gradually introduce change that starts small and eventually becomes all encompassing.

But before we go on, perhaps I should explain what I mean by 'change everything'. Why do you need to change everything if all you want to do is get a little more energy?

Let's look at one example and use that as a microcosmic example of why it doesn't work to try and change one aspect of your health and lifestyle in a vacuum.

Why You've Failed to Get Into Shape

If you're like an awful lot of people, then at some point you have probably tried to get into better shape. That might mean you joined a gym, or perhaps you paid for a training program to get written for you.

And if you're like an awful lot of people, then you may well have failed to stick at the training program or to see the results you wanted.

Why is that?

Probably, it comes down to the simple fact that the training program was too ambitious. Very often, a training program will involve working out three, four or five times a week at a gym. As a standard rule, workouts will be somewhere between 40-60 minutes.

So that's immediately 4-5 hours of extra time that you need to take away from your current working week.

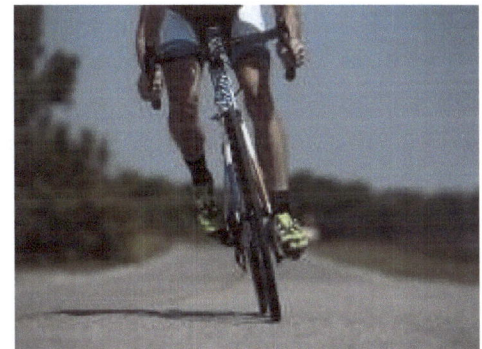

Then there's the fact that you need to travel to and from the gym. This can take anything from 10 minutes each way to 30 minutes. Then there's showering and then there's the amount of extra *washing* you create and the fact that you need to pack for the gym.

So what you're really doing is taking about 10 hours out of your working week. That's huge.

And more to the point, these are ten *exhausting* hours.

And that's before we've even considered the amount of work we're expected to do in the kitchen: we're supposed to be transforming our diets to be low calorie (meaning low energy) and we're supposed to shop for the food, cook the food, wash up afterward...

And it's all *stressful* too. Cooking can be stressful and so can spending all that extra money on the gym, on the food, on the petrol... it's just too much!

There's a good chance that the very reason you're not exercising and getting enough activity right now is that you're too tired half of the time. This is why so many of us let ourselves get into bad shape to begin with. It's why we turn to junk food. And it's why we struggle to stick at new goals.

In short, we're already doing as much as we can.

So again, the problem here is energy. Energy management is more important than time management by far when it comes to exercise so really you need to focus on getting more energy or managing what you have better. So next let's look at what's sapping energy in your life. For many of us diet comes into play here and eating lots of junk food can certainly prevent us from feeling our very best and healthiest. So that needs to be changed.

More important though is work. If you are coming home from work stressed, then you're going to have very little energy for throwing yourself into a workout. Likewise, stress from other sources, such as your finances or relationships can also have a negative impact on your ability to train. So you need to fix that too.

There are practical considerations too like finances (staying in shape can be expensive!) and like space if you're training at home (which is a good shout for most people). Even if you're not training from home, having a tidy apartment, flat or house to come home to can make all the difference in terms of your energy and how you feel; it means you have one less thing to do at the end of the day (tidying up in this case). Likewise, looking good will fill you with energy and confidence too which will translate to a better mood and more energy to attack workouts. A lot of energy is linked with mood, as we'll see later in this book.

Then of course those other things do also come into play: time, motivation and the right program.

The point I'm making is that picking a training program and pledging to stick at it just doesn't work unless you're also looking at what has been holding you back so far. Right now you probably fill your time with activity as much as you can and then crash on the sofa because you're out of steam. If you had the energy to work out, then you'd already be working out. You're not, because you don't. So don't come up with an unrealistic 5-day workout plan until you've looked at the rest of your life – including your physical energy, happiness and mental discipline. You have to change everything if you want to get into great shape.

And as you'll see, this then makes changes in the rest of your life. Working out will *give* you more energy. And when you get more energy, you will find you start to perform better at work. This will be helped by the fact that you now look and feel more confident and attractive filling out that suit/pencil skirt with a more toned physique.

Working less means you'll have more energy to train.

Training means you'll have more energy to do better at work.

And these kinds of two-way relationships exist throughout your entire lifestyle.

Deciding What Matters

Your lifestyle is self-sustaining then and everything you do is supporting that lifestyle and making it harder for you to change. So where can you possibly start?

As mentioned, one of the key things to think about is energy management and planning. Just knowing that you have a finite amount of energy throughout the day and then making decisions on that basis.

And this brings us to our first, super important tip:

If you're going to introduce something big into your life, then you need to remove something else.

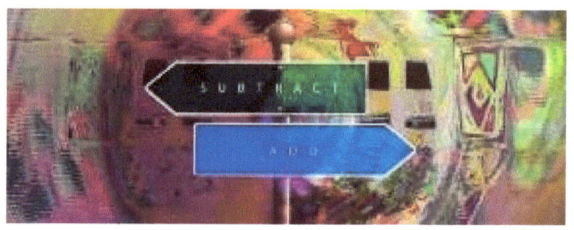

This sounds like a big deal and many of us will be resistant to it at first. But it's also true.

If you're going to try and exert yourself for 30 minutes after work every day, then you need to find a way to *save* 30 minutes of both time *and* energy. Getting up 30 minutes earlier will give you more time. But perhaps going to bed 1 hour earlier the night before can give you some more of the energy you need.

Or perhaps you just make the decision to save energy by going out a *little* less. If you have a weekly pub trip, then consider cutting that out (especially seeing as alcohol will sap your energy in the long term). If you have a very busy social calendar, perhaps consider seeing one friend less. That sounds harsh but life is all about making tough decisions.

Or maybe you'd rather cut out one of your more tiring hobbies/extracurricular activities?

Again, it's hard and it seems cold. But the simple fact of the matter is that every action needs an equal and opposite reaction. You can't pull extra time out of thin air.

But that's what is going to bring us to our next chapter and a somewhat more appealing sounding alternative: finding lots of little ways to save more time and more energy throughout the day. This is where the concept of kaizen comes in. If you can save a little energy on the way to work, save a little energy in the morning, save a little energy doing the dishes... well then you might just have a bit more to 'spend' doing the things you love and the things that are important to you.

Chapter Three: The Small Changes That Will Supercharge Your Energy Levels

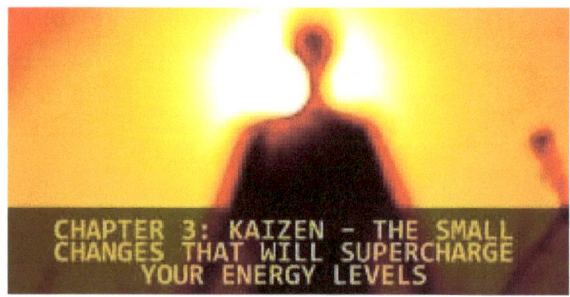

To spend more time doing the things you love – and engaging in activities that will actually *boost* your energy further – you need to find ways to save time throughout the day. That way, you can introduce new things to your routine without feeling like you're being pushed too far. This will also help you to recharge and relax by having some time spare, which will ultimately help you to be even more focussed, productive and creative at work!

Tidy

Believe it or not, tidying your home makes a massive difference to your energy levels, your confidence and therefore your ability to stick to your training. Think of your home as an extension of your state of mind – if you're very stressed, your home is more likely to look a mess. If your home is a mess, you'll be more stressed.

So what's the easiest way to keep your home tidier and to give yourself more mental clarity and space? Actually it's to get ruthless and just throw things out. Got a box of junk on the dresser that you haven't looked in for a year?

Get rid of it. Got 20 ornaments or knick-knacks on every surface? Throw out half of those dust-collectors (at least!). This may sound extreme but simply having more space, even just seeing out the corner of your eye that there's space under the bed, can make a huge difference to your state of mind. The lack of clutter makes it easier for your mind and body to unwind. Clutter and mess literally causes you to produce norepinephrine, cortisol and other stress hormones, which can end up leaving you feeling completely spent unless you can do something about it.

This is particularly useful when you consider that it will also make tidying up much easier in future. Now you'll be able to clean surfaces by wiping a wet cloth, without having to remove lots of items from around your home. Finding things will be easier and generally, you'll find you have more time and energy as a result.

Oh and when you remove 50% of your ornaments, you'll be left with a much higher 'average quality' of things left on display. This actually makes your home look much wealthier and more impressive, because there's no longer the less impressive stuff to detract from the truly great stuff...

Shop Online

Most of us will do at least one – probably two – big shops every week. This involves driving to the supermarket, walking around the aisles, loading up our shopping carts or baskets, wrestling with other customers and then loading up our bags and carrying them to the car.

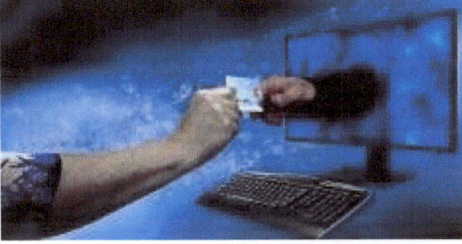

That's a heck of a lot of effort!

Not to mention the fact that when you shop like this, you have no idea of the budget or the precise amount you're spending.

If you want to perform optimally at work the next day, then spending your evenings hunting around supermarkets with screaming kids is not the way to do it...

And so it actually makes a lot more sense to shop online. Set up a selection of items that you want to buy – you can even do this on your lunch break – and then have them delivered each week with a few variations to keep your meals interesting. You just saved yourself 1-3 hours a week and those hours would have involved a lot of exertion.

That's enough time to work on a book!

Automate the Cleaning

Back to cleaning and tidying!

Because even with a very well organized home and minimal clutter, you're still going to find yourself needing to clean from time to time, meaning that you're not either relaxing and recuperating *or* doing things you enjoy.

But many of these types of work can be avoided or at least minimized too. For example, you could take away the need to wash up after eating by simply using your dishwasher more instead of hand washing dishes. Sick of spending lots of time vacuuming? Then how about getting a robotic vacuum cleaner? Ironing taking too long? How about buying no-iron clothes!

If you want to go even further, then you could consider ordering ready-made meal deliveries to come to your door (as long as they adhere to the diet recommendations we're going to go into) and you could look into getting a house maid service to help you keep your home in top shape.

In short, there's really no reason to spend your hard-earned time and energy sweeping the floor and cooking. It might seem 'lazy' but it really isn't if you're using that time to do other fun and useful things.

Do you think Obama spends his time washing dishes? Richard Branson? Do you think they'd have time to run their empires if they did? Do you think they'd have the energy? As you may have noticed, some of these trade-offs require the spending of money, but why not? If you have the money to spend, why not trade dollars for more time and energy?

Stretching and Foam Rolling

Stretching is something I never used to bother with until I heard someone point out how much younger it made them feel once they got their flexibility back. And it makes sense – if you come home from work and covered in aches and pains – then of course you're not going to be brimming with energy! And most of us lead lifestyles that make us all the more stiff and achy. If you spend a huge amount of your time sitting at a desk, then this is going to do nothing short of destroying your health. Sitting for long stretches is terrible for your heart (because you're not using it, basically), while it also causes certain muscles to shorten and tighten, while others elongate and become weaker. Among other things, this can risk causing an 'anterior pelvic tilt' where your pelvis is actually pulled forward at the front, making your buttocks protrude and hurting your back.

Doing *everything* is harder if this is the state you're moving around in!

Start and end your workouts with stretching. Use dynamic stretching before working out to warm up the muscles and get the blood flowing. Use static stretching post-workout to cool down.

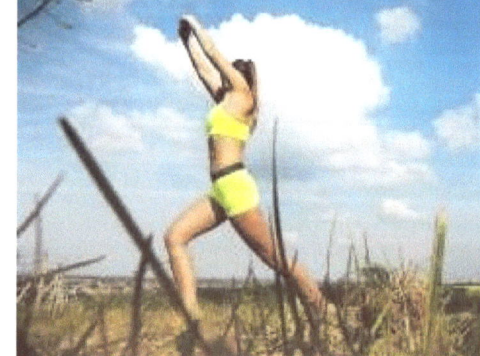

Foam rolling can help workout knots that may have developed over time. Also known as Self-Myofascial Release (SMR), massaging your muscles by rolling them over a foam cylinder can increase joint range of motion by breaking down fascia scar tissue that forms from muscle repair.

Commuting

One of the most tiring parts of the day for so many of us is the commute – and there are countless reasons for this. Not only does commuting often mean you need to get up an hour or more before you would otherwise have to, but it also means you need to push yourself onto a crowded bus or train with lots of other people, or sit in a traffic jam cursing (which just increases your stress level and drains your energy).

When you've just spent a whole day being shouted at or dealing with work responsibilities, this can be too much for us to handle sometimes.

There are plenty of solutions though. One is to look into flex-time. Ask your boss if you can come in an hour earlier and leave an hour earlier – it may mean you miss rush hour and it shouldn't hurt your productivity. It also means you'll have an extra hour or so to yourself at the start of the day where you can be much more productive.

Another option is to consider a car-pool. This way, you can get a lift into work every other day, making life much easier for you. The stress is now split in half, at least, as is the cost of fuel.

And if there's nothing else you can do, then think about the ways you can make work the journey a little more relaxing and a little less stressful. This might mean reading a great book with headphones and some good music, or it might mean napping to get even more energy in!

Don't overlook telecommuting or working from home. Depending on the type of work you do, you may be able to do it at least a day or two per week from the comfort of your home. Without a commute or distractions in the office, many people actually get a lot more done working from home.

Chapter Four: How to Enhance Your Sleep to Enhance Your Day

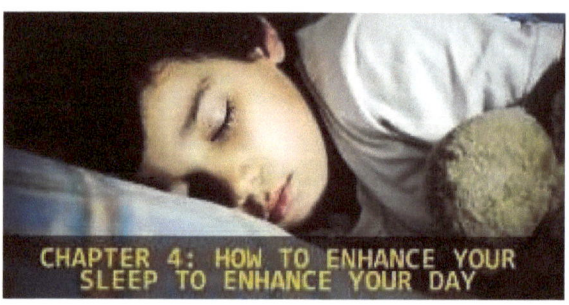

Forget smart drugs, the single best way to enhance your cognitive powers and become more focused is to get more sleep.

And forget supplements, the single best way to accelerate your muscle gains and improve your strength is to get more sleep.

There are countless articles out there that detail 'life hacks' and other strategies you can use to sleep better. These range between lying on spikey mats (which is nonsense), to taking ZMA (which doesn't do much), to eating honey before bed (which might just be helpful but is negligible).

More efficient then is to look at some small, simple changes – six as a matter-of-fact - you can make to your routine that will have a major impact on the quality and quantity of your sleep. There's that 'kaizen' again!

Number one: Take a hot shower or bath before bed. This helps to encourage the production of growth hormone and melatonin and it also helps to relax the muscles – far more effectively than taking valerian root. As your body cools down, you'll sink into a much deeper and more restorative sleep and you'll also save yourself time in the morning.

Number two: Open the window a-jar. We sleep much better when our environment is slightly cool. Let some cool air into your room but make sure you can keep warm with your duvet or coverlet.

Number three: Go for a run or walk in the morning that day. Getting more exercise helps you sleep better, as does getting fresh air and vitamin D. You can also supplement with vitamin D in the morning – if you live in an area where it is cloudy a lot, then there's a good chance you're deficient.

Number four: Take half an hour or even just 15 minutes before bed to wind down and do some reading. Avoid looking at mobile screens or computers if possible, as the light from these increases cortisol production. I experimented with wearing blue-blocking shades before bed for a while but truth be told, you look like a nob and it's pretty impractical – especially if you're in a relationship. Taking a little while out to 'unwind' will help you forget the stresses of the day while getting your body into a good 'sleep mode'. To save time, do your reading while taking your bath.

Number five: Most important of all is simply to prioritize your sleep and to give it the attention it deserves. Stop watching YouTube videos until 2am in the morning and start getting into a sleep routine.

Number six: Of course you also need to look after the environment you're sleeping in. Comfortable pajamas and bed covers, along with curtains that actually block out the light and an absence of blinking LEDs will make a huge difference.

Waking Up Full of Energy and Vitality

Meanwhile, I highly recommend investing in some kind of 'daylight alarm' (such as those made by Lumie). These are designed to emit a light that is more similar to sunlight in terms of the wavelength and will come on gradually as it approaches the time you 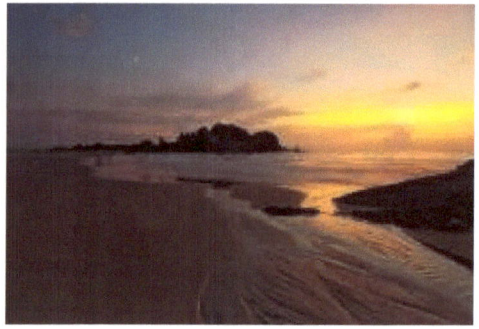 set the alarm. This then gradually rouses you out of sleep and if all goes well, you'll wake naturally before the alarm goes off. As a result, you'll feel significantly more awake and well rested. Even if it takes the alarm to wake you though, you'll be waking up in a light environment from a much lighter state of sleep. You feel far less 'sleep inertia' and you'll really notice the difference when you're forced to wake up without it. This is especially effective for those who struggle with SAD (Seasonal Affective Disorder). Trust me, this is one change that will really make a highly noticeable difference.

Just think about the difference you're now making: previously, you were sleeping deeply at which point a loud alarm would suddenly startle you awake. This would jolt you out of sleep with a start and you'd wake up into a pitch black room and have to drag yourself out of bed.

Instead, you're now coming around gently, waking up gradually and naturally as the room gets lighter and then being nudged over the edge by the actual alarm. And when you open your eyes, the room is already light and you're already ready to go!

Get Up on Time Every Time

For those who struggle to get out of bed without hitting the 'snooze' button, a daylight alarm can help. If you need a little extra help, then try waking up in 'stages'. Instead of forcing yourself to leap out of bed, agree that you'll just prop yourself up into a more upright position and turn on the light when the alarm sounds. If you must hit snooze then that's fine, but just once! The second time it goes off, you're then going to grab a book, your phone or something else that will prevent you from dozing off again. Absent mindedly look through this. Then, you should find you're awake enough to get up. Getting up slowly is not only healthier, it's much easier to do when you're feeling low on will-power.

Why You Feel Ill in the Morning

If you find you still can't wake up effectively in the morning, then it may be that you're struggling with a number of potential issues. If you have a scratchy throat or you feel ill, then below you'll find some possible causes and solutions:

• Allergy – You can develop hay fever at any age and symptoms that are unnoticeable during the day can be much worse at night when you've been breathing in dander or pollen all night. Unfortunately, most antihistamines will leave you feeling groggy too, so you'll need to find another way to clean your environment.

• Mold – Mold poisoning can lead to a number of unpleasant short term and long term effects. If you have mycotoxin-producing black mold it can even give you asthma or eczema. Even just breathing in mold spores from less harmful types can leave you with a scratchy throat and a poor night's sleep. If you notice the air smelling damp, then consider calling in a mold remediation company – it could be behind the walls or under the floorboards.

• Dehydration – It's common to get dehydrated during the night. Make sure you drink enough before you fall asleep and have some water to hand. If you struggle with this one, you may want to consider trying chia seeds which absorb several times their mass' worth of water.

• Low blood sugar – Breakfast is so named because you are 'breaking your fast'. As you can imagine, going 10 hours without eating can leave you a little groggy so it's possible you're struggling with low blood sugar. Something that is thought to help this is a spoon of honey, which contains both slow release and fast release sugar, providing you with a steady supply of energy through the night.

This might seem like a bit of a random tangent but it really isn't – many of us wake up in the morning feeling sub-par but aren't quite sure why. Often it comes down to factors in the environment or in your overall health like these and as we've seen, it should be relatively easy to solve them in many cases!

CBT for Getting to Sleep

Finally, if you struggle getting to sleep because you can't stop your mind racing, then address the way you are thinking about sleep.

There's a lot more to learn about CBT (Cognitive Behavorial Therapy) and it really is a fantastic tool but for now all you need to know is that it involves changing the way you think about a problem. In this case, you're going to stop putting pressure on yourself to sleep – if you feel stressed that you're not asleep yet, then you'll work yourself up and be far less likely to be able to drift off!

Instead of getting frustrated then, focus on using the opportunity to just relax and enjoy lying down to have a think/feel free from the pressures of the day. Even if you're just relaxing, this will still offer you some recuperative benefit. What you'll find though, is that the moment you manage to enjoy 'just relaxing', you'll fall asleep. Don't force yourself to drift off, that's an oxymoron; just get comfortable, enjoy the moment and let your body take care of the rest when you really need to drift off.

Chapter Five: Ride the Tide

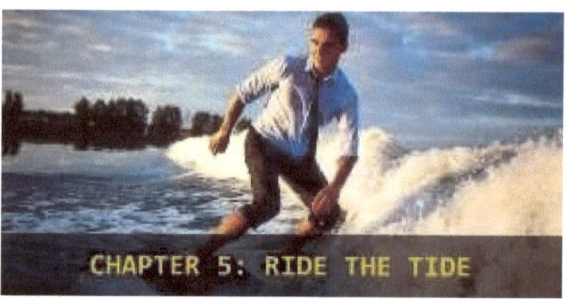

CHAPTER 5: RIDE THE TIDE

Our energy levels come in ebbs and flows and we are all beholden to this natural 'cycle'. At certain points during the day you will feel energetic and at others, you'll feel listless and exhausted. Instead of trying to force your body to be energetic when you need it to be and tired when you want to go to bed, try choosing activities based on how you feel.

This is the idea of 'riding the tide'. Again, it's about acknowledging that there *is* a limit to how much energy you can utilize in any given day and planning your activities out smartly as a result of and in tune with that ebb and flow.

In this chapter, we're going to look at the energy cycles that your body goes through in any given day. We'll explore what *causes* those energy cycles and we'll look at how you can actually influence them in order to help them align more usefully with the activities that you need to commit yourself to in any given day.

Why Your Body Has Energy Cycles

Let's start by addressing why your body goes through energy cycles in the first place.

And the answer comes down to evolution and survival. We have adapted to function this way, because it helps us to survive in a dangerous environment and to manage energy levels in the wild. The problem is that we're no longer in the wild and we now need energy at different times.

Ultimately, these energy systems work by splitting us into two states. These are:

- Anabolic
- Catabolic

An anabolic state is also referred to as 'rest and digest'. This is when we're relaxed, happy and able to just switch off and chill. During this time, the body has plenty of fuel (energy) and it is able to send that fuel where it's needed to help us repair muscle, lay down memories and restore ourselves during sleep.

Conversely, a catabolic state is also referred to as 'fight or flight'. This is when we're either in danger, or we're starving. Either our blood sugar is low, or we are being faced by a predator or a threat (stress). Either way, the reality is that our bodies need to *act* to keep us alive and thus we start burning fat and even muscle to provide fuel.

Of course you're not always asleep or scared for your life, but you are always teetering slightly *more* to one of these extremes or the other. When you wake up in the morning, your blood sugar levels are low and this is what causes you to wake up. You've been fasting and your body is now running on empty, which triggers the release of stress hormones like cortisol.

When you've just eaten meanwhile, your body receives the signal that it is satiated and that the blood is filled with sugar. Thus it releases insulin to extract that sugar and it releases serotonin which makes you feel good. That serotonin eventually converts to melatonin – the sleep hormone – and the body is able to rest and use all that good stuff to help repair our bodies.

This cycle of anabolic/catabolic, stop/go continues all throughout the day. It is also closely linked with our 'circadian rhythm', which is our sleep-wake cycle.

Psychologists have studies our circadian rhythms extensively and what they've discovered is that they are determined by two main factors: 'external zeitgebers' (time givers) and 'internal pacemakers'. In short, we listen to the cues from our body, as well as the cues from the world around us – like the amount of light and social cues.

This is why the daylight lamp I mentioned in the last chapter is so valuable – the light stimulates the release of cortisol and nitric oxide, both of which help the brain to wake up. It's also why it's so important that we get a few minutes to let our 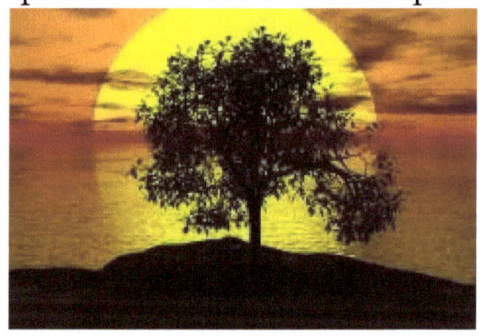 bodies cool down in the evening without unnatural light. Having a vitamin D supplement also helps – our bodies produce vitamin D when they receive direct sunlight.

Another factor that contributes to us needing to sleep, is the build-up of two substances in the brain: adenosine and pro-inflammatory cytokines.

Adenosine is the main by-product of the brain's energy process. That is to say, when your brain cells are working, they're constantly creating adenosine as well. The harder you think and the more active you are, the more adenosine builds up. And as it builds up, it suppresses activity – making it harder and harder for us to concentrate and contributing to 'brain fog'. Eventually, this becomes too much and we need to sleep to clear it.

Meanwhile, pro-inflammatory cytokines cause brain inflammation. These too build up as a result of our immune system working overtime and they're highest in number when we feel sick. This is why we feel tired, groggy and full of brain fog when we're ill (which is partly our body's way of telling us to hit the hay).

All this means that there are points in the day when we will feel our most awake and points when we feel our most asleep. Most of us will experience a serious crash around 4am and 4pm. We sleep deepest at 4am and we struggle to focus on work at 4pm. The afternoon time is the ideal time to schedule a break then. Better yet, if you can move your working day forward an hour, then you can come home at the point when you're feeling most tired!

How to Manage Your Energy Levels

While it's a good idea to fit your work schedule around your energy ebbs and flows , it would of course be slightly more convenient if you could alternatively fit your energy around your work schedule. Fortunately, there are some things you can do to alter your rhythms and help yourself to feel more energetic right when you need to.

One simple way to do this is to think about when and how you're going to eat. Remember: when we eat, it stimulates the sudden release of sugar into the blood, which can result in us feeling very tired and lethargic immediately afterward. This is great an hour or so before bed (giving you time to digest) but it's not so useful if you were planning on being useful that evening.

A simple example of this is what happens when you sit down and eat dinner on the couch in the evening. Any hopes you might have had of being productive at this point are practically thrown out the window. So instead, if you wanted to tidy the house, try doing it *before* you eat, while your body is still flooding you full of wakefulness hormones.

Another way to control your energy levels through your diet is to think about *what* you want to eat. A big mistake is to eat simple carbohydrates, which are things like cake, like bread and like white pasta. These release sugar quickly into the blood stream, which results in a sudden energy 'high'. However, as we now know, that will be released by a sudden 'crash' when the sugar is taken up and the brain releases melatonin to put you in a restorative mode.

The solution to this is to try and keep your blood sugar at a slightly more stable and level point throughout the day. In theory, this should provide you with a steady flow of energy, while at the same time avoiding sugar crashes or sudden spikes in energy.

To do this, you can focus on getting more energy from both complex carbohydrates (carbohydrates that are slower to digest, normally including more fiber and fat) as well as fats (which also digest slowly in the gut).

Both these methods will provide a consistent level of energy as you go about your day and may also have other health benefits – potentially reducing inflammation. We'll discuss this more in the 'diet' section of the book.

Changing the order of your food – even just by shifting everything forward an hour – can help to change the order and length of your cycles. In fact, when travelling abroad to different time zones, many people will utilize a system of changing their diet to readjust their circadian rhythms and body clocks.

Another tip is to consider taking power naps. This is something that some people have a lot of success with but there is a trick to it which will once again involve thinking in terms of cycles. This main objective is to avoid waking up *during* a sleep cycle. Sleep cycles tend to last about 90 minutes but it takes 20 minutes to enter the first heavy stage of sleep. Sleeping for just 10 minutes can be a great way to get a quick energy boost then, while sleeping for 90 minutes should provide a deeper sleep while helping you to avoid waking up during 'SWS' (slow wave sleep) and experiencing high levels of sleep inertia as a result.

Finding a Routine for Optimum Performance

The key thing to take away from this, is that you need to consider the role of your body in your energy levels. What you eat, what time you sleep and even the light outside can all affect your energy levels and your mood.

Even the temperature can have a huge impact – if you are in a cold room, this will increase your production of adrenaline and norepinephrine, thereby making you feel more alert.

Conversely, if you're in a warm space, then you'll feel more relaxed and sleepy and may find it harder to stay awake.

Note that we are more creative when we're relaxed. This allows our mind to wander and it's when the mind wanders that it can form novel connections between concepts, thereby creating entirely new ideas.

You can even split your work into ebbs and flows this way then – dividing it between periods of creativity where you come up with new ideas and directions and periods of productivity where you go full steam ahead to work as hard as possible.

Which of course is a simple way of saying – you need to take breaks!

Chapter Six: The Devastating Effect of Stress

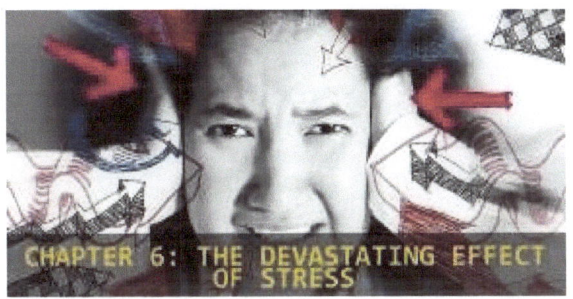

This brings us nicely to the topic of stress, another critical element of our wake/sleep cycle and our energy.

Remember, stress is what triggers the 'fight or flight' response. Stress is the response to a perceived threat and/or low blood sugar.

It's worth noting this right away because if you're feeling hungry *and* you have a deadline, then you're going to be more stressed out than you would be trying to tackle the same issue while you were asleep!

A little stress is a good thing. A little stress is what we call 'eustress' and this is what motivates us to focus and to be productive. Moreover, a little stress helps us stay awake and alert and to focus on whatever it is we're doing.

The problem is when we have too much stress, or when this stress lasts too long. Remember, we're supposed to go through cycles where we switch between 'awake and alert' and 'relaxed and calm'.

So what do you think happens if you're *highly* 'awake and alert' for 8 hours straight without a break? That's right: you come home and absolutely *collapse* in a heap because you're 100% spent.

And there is a good physiological reason for this too. When you exert yourself, you are producing hormones that keep your energy levels high. These include adrenaline and norepinephrine, which keep your heart beating faster and help you concentrate and focus.

The problem is, that there's only so much of these neurochemicals that we can produce. Eventually we run out, which causes something called 'adrenal fatigue'. In this state, we will experience incredibly low energy, low mood and low motivation!

Ask yourself: what is the single most tiring part of your day?

It's probably work.

And this is because you have been producing these 'go, go, go' hormones for 8 hours straight – which is entirely unnatural. That much focus meanwhile increases the amount of adenosine and the amount of cytokines. Worse still, is that your *body* is not working at all, meaning that you're going to be feeling exhausted and spent despite not having had any useful exercise.

What's more, being constantly 'on' throughout the day is a good way to cause health problems. These cycles are here for a reason. When you eat and then go straight back into work, the large amount of stress actually suppresses your digestion.

Remember: stress in the wild was often associated with danger and we don't want to be digesting when we're meant to be running!

Meanwhile, your immune system is also suppressed – which is why you're much more likely to become ill when "overstressed".

And remember what we said in the last chapter about creativity? Well stress is the mortal enemy of creativity. In fact, stress causes the prefrontal cortex – the smart and 'creative' part of our brain – to shut down entirely. This leads to mistakes and means you're not going to be performing your best at all.

If you allow this to go on long enough, the worst-case scenario is that it leads to depression and/or serious illness. The best-case scenario is that you'll spend your evenings staring blankly into space with no will power, motivation or energy to do anything.

How to Prevent Stress From Destroying Your Energy Levels

So what can you do to prevent stress from robbing you of your energy?

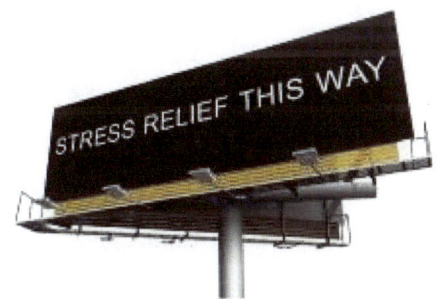

The first key is to make sure you are taking time out and that you make this a *mental* break as well as a physical one.

In other words, take a break from thinking about work and instead try reading, or perhaps going for a nice, quiet stroll. This is another reason why many health and fitness experts recommend going for a walk during your lunch break. Just be sure to leave enough time at the end to eat (your healthy brown bag lunch you brought from home). Either way, you should focus on thinking about anything *other* than work.

An even better idea is to practice some stress management techniques. CBT (Cognitive Behavioral Therapy) is a great method to this end, as is meditation. Either way, if you can go through your working day and remain calm and relatively unfazed even when everything seems to be going wrong, you'll find that the entire day seems *much* less tiring and thus you arrive home with far more energy to spend being productive or just having fun. It also means you'll have more energy at work the next day to be more productive.

And finally? If work is repeatedly taking it all out of you and you can't find a way to get the balance right... you should quit.

Again, this sounds extreme. But if your work is that tiring or that stressful, then it will only continue to undermine your enjoyment of other activities and eventually start to take a toll on your health. Your health and happiness should *always* come first and there's no reason that anyone ever must stay stuck in a job that is placing so much strain on them.

Chapter Seven: Training for Energy

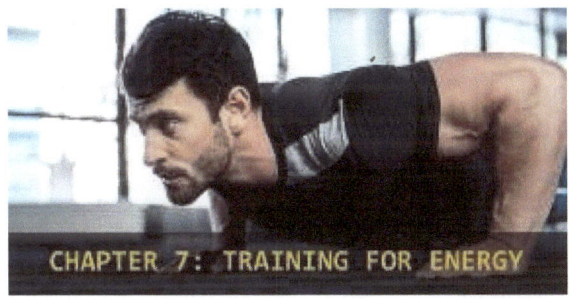

The first reason for this is that exercise will help you to enhance your cellular efficiency. Inside each of your cells are tiny little 'energy factories' called mitochondria. These are what take the energy (glucose) from your food and convert it into something used (ATP). They're also what break that ATP down to release the energy that drives muscle contractions, deep thought and *breathing*.

As we get older, the number of mitochondria in our system depletes. But when you're a young kid, you have loads of them and they're functioning much more efficiently.

So if you ever wondered why all Grandpa does is sleep, while little Timmy rushes around the house all day on a sugar-high, that would be why.

But when you exercise, you boost the function and number of your mitochondria. This doesn't just help you to perform better in athletic activities – it also helps you to *think* better and to wake up more alert so that you can get more done.

That's only *one* way in which exercise will boost your productivity. Another powerful effect comes from improved cardio fitness, circulation and blood pressure.

In short, using your heart a lot will make stronger, thus allowing you to better pump blood around your body and providing you with oxygen, nutrients etc. The best form of exercise for this benefit is steady state cardio. Running long distance gives your heart's 'left ventricle' time to enlarge and that means you can pump more blood around more easily.

But any form of exercise will help you increase your VO2 max, your resting heartrate and your energy levels.

Exercise is also *super good* for your brain and will encourage more brain plasticity, improving your sleep. Getting rid of fat will make you lighter, meaning you spend less energy moving around.

In short, if you can exercise, you will perform *much* better than ever before.

The only problem?

If you're currently not exercising at all, then you'll find it hard to start. Which is why I'm happy to introduce the 'QUICK' routine to solve that problem...

A Basic Training Program to Boost Your Energy

The most important thing to start with is a simple training program that you just *stick at.* This is where all these self-help books and online training programs have gotten things a bit twisted.

It is very misguided when you see the people who walk around the gym with elaborate training programs and queueing for machines even before they've developed a basic level of fitness.

It's even more misguided when people tell themselves that they haven't started working out yet because they need to 'find the right training program'.

Want to lose weight? Then you might have taken a quick look online to find advice. Some people will be telling you to cut your carbs, others will be telling you to count calories and not worry about carbs. Others will tell you to eat *more* carbs and cut the fat! Meanwhile, do you do steady state cardio (jogging) or do you try HIIT (High Intensity Interval Training)? It's all a lot to pick from!

At this point though, it really doesn't matter. All that matters is that you are doing *something*. If you aren't already training, then get training right now on a regular basis – don't wait until you've finished this book!

Don't focus on improving your health or getting abs (though we'll touch on that down the bottom) – just focus on getting good at training and actually sticking to a routine.

Anything is better than nothing and you don't need to worry about training 'wrong' – your body is incredibly adaptable.

So here's a very simple training routine you can use to just 'start' getting into shape:

The QUICK Program

1. Press-Ups (Push-Ups) to Failure (keep going until you can't do anymore, remember the number and beat it next time)
2. Pull-Ups to Failure
3. Kettlebell Swings to Failure (use a weight that allows you to do about 30 to begin with)

There is no pause in between each exercise and you should treat this like a circuit. Ideally you should aim to do 3-5 rounds of each exercise with one minute rest after the swings, but if you only have time to do one that's okay. Remember: *it's better to do something than nothing*. The second piece of advice - *it is never too late to start*. If you have just 5 minutes at the end of the day, then just doing the press-ups is fine.

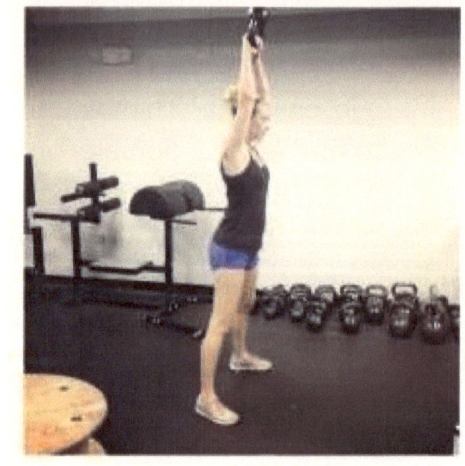

Perform the press-ups fast and keep your body rigid as you do. Make sure you go all the way down and back up for each rep.

Look for the Iron Gym for a pull-up bar that fits into a doorframe without needing screws. This will set you back about $25.

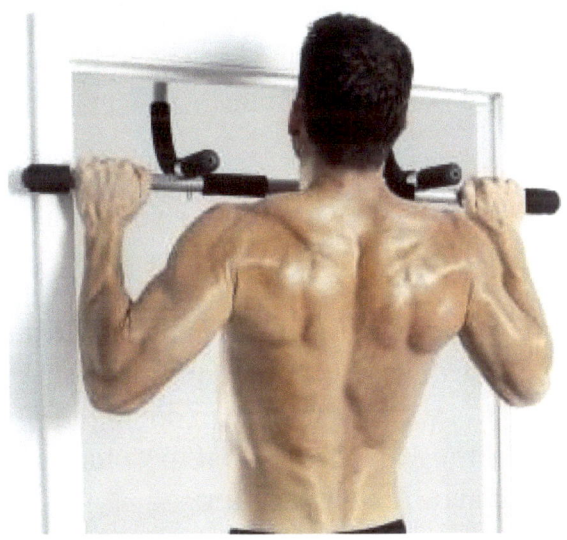

If you don't have a kettlebell set, you can buy one online for about $30.

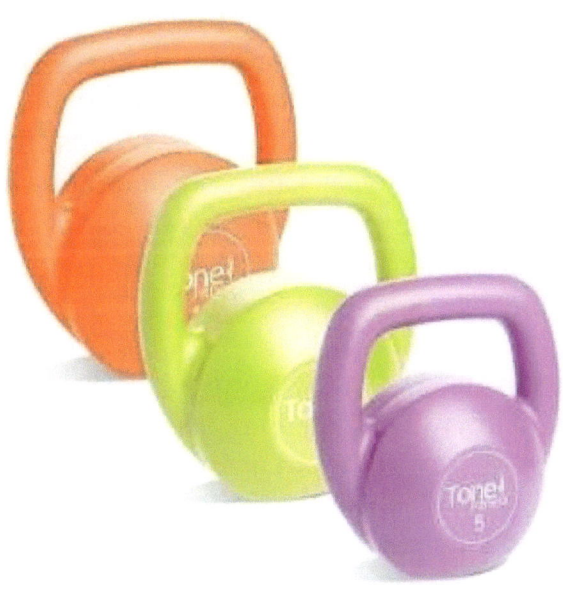

For less than $60, you can set yourself up with a gym at home to do the QUICK workout. It is a lot less money than a gym membership and saves time in the end by not having to go to the gym and then back home.

If that's still off the cards, then you can replace the kettlebell swings with jack-in-the-box reps. Here you squat down, then explode up and splay your arms and legs apart.

With all these you are starting by going to failure and then aiming to increase or maintain that number each time you come to do the workout. So if you can do 30 press-ups right now, you'll be aiming to increase that to 31 tomorrow. In a year, you'll be maybe doing 70 or 100.

Try to do this at *least* four times a week to see the real results.

Why the QUICK Routine is Effective

This routine is the 'only necessary exercise' because it offers some cardio benefit when practiced with intensity and it offers resistance training too for all the major muscle groups. The push-ups train the pecs, shoulders, triceps and core, the pull-ups train the lats, biceps and core and the swings train the hamstrings, quads and lower back (erector spinae). Overall, this is about as close to a 'full body' routine as you're going to get in just three moves.

But what really makes this routine effective is the simplicity. You can use it anywhere, you don't need much equipment and it's completely flexible and adaptable. If you can only do one round then that's fine – and there's never really an excuse not to be able to do 5 minutes of exercise.

The great thing is though, once you've done one round you'll probably find you have the energy and determination to complete two more.

With its simplicity, the QUICK routine is designed very much for beginners and is not intended for those who want to build big muscle or crushing strength. If you're new to training then starting out with something to improve your general fitness and muscle tone is very important.

How to Get Abs

By the way, the QUICK program is also ideal for helping you to get abs.

Getting visible abs is mainly about diet with the aim being to reduce your body fat percentage to sub 10% thus making the six-pack visible underneath. We'll be looking at that later in this section. This is aided though by CV (cardiovascular)training 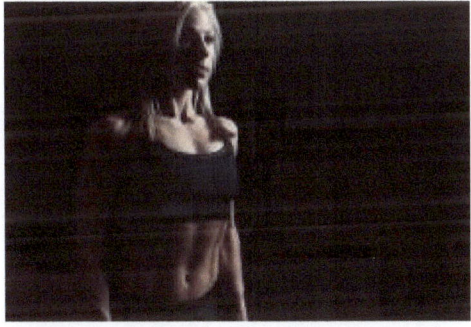 and once you start doing kettlebell swings and push-ups for reps of 100, this will be quite a cardio-intensive routine.

The other thing people forget though is their transverse abdominis. This is the band of muscle around your mid-section that acts to hold in your stomach and internal organs, as well as to support your lower spine during lifts. Crucially, this is what makes your abs *flat* and that in turn is what makes them look good. Push-ups require you to keep your whole body rigid and this is the *perfect* way to ensure you are strengthening the transverse abdominis.

So do the QUICK workout regularly and with intensity, and you should start to find your abs showing. Hopefully that will offer some motivation to some readers!

How to Write Goals and Increase Adherence

Don't approach your training with the goal of trying to lose 'X amount of weight' or gain 'X amount of muscle'. Why? Because that's not completely within your control. If you give yourself such a defined set of goals, then you'll find things get in the way and you become frustrated as you realize you may fail. Instead, give yourself a simple and clearly defined goal that is *completely* within your control.

For instance: do the QUICK workout four times a week. That's it. Your *only* goal. This is something you will succeed or fail at and you get to try anew every week. If you do that long enough, you will find that the 'bigger goals' (like weight loss and muscle mass) take care of themselves.

Focusing on long term goals is also a bad idea because it leads to training that's much less enjoyable. Try to forget about why you're going to the gym and just *enjoy* being there so that it's its own reward. When I'm really low on motivation I just go and hit the heavy bag which I love.

Priming

A little tip – if you're feeling very low on energy and can't get the motivation to hit the gym, then try watching something that motivates you. The *Rocky 4* training montage tends to do the trick for me. This is called 'priming' in psychology and you can use the technique in other areas of your life too. Need to sit down to do some coding?

Try watching a snippet of *The Social Network* or *Iron Man* and see if that puts you in your 'genius mode' mentality.

It sounds like a small matter but when we feel driven to do something, it actually makes a big difference to our energy levels. This triggers a similar sort of neurochemical/hormonal response to eustress because you're telling your body and mind that what you're doing *matters* and is important. Remind yourself why you're doing what you're doing and you can put yourself in that waking mode more easily.

Chapter Eight: Fuel

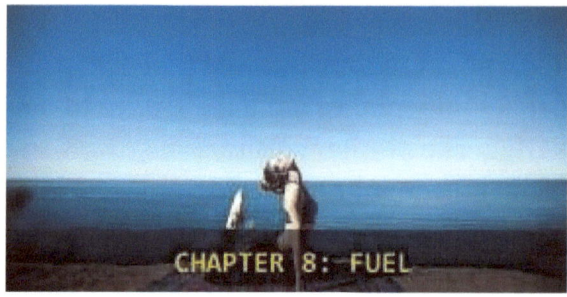

When you want to give your car more energy, what do you do? You fill it with gas!

And of course it only stands to reason that you need to do the exact same thing when you're giving *yourself* more fuel.

Well, not the *exact* same thing. You're not filling yourself with gas – but with fuel yes!

We've already seen that one of the most important ways to manage your energy levels is to think harder about your carbs and your timing with them. By consuming more complex carbs – like oats – and more fats – like avocado – you can provide yourself with a steady supply of energy throughout the day.

But there's more to it than that too of course. What's also very important is simply to make sure that you're providing yourself with *enough* calories and that you're spacing your food out enough. This is critical just to ensure there's a steady supply of energy while you're going about your business. This is also why going extremely low carb may be a mistake: studies show us that you see a reduction in IQ when you go *too* low carb. The simple reason is that there isn't enough energy for the brain to function optimally.

Why Nutrients Matter

So food is fuel but it's also much more than that. Food is also what provides your body with the raw materials it needs to help you function optimally. And when you functional optimally, you have more energy!

Nutrients are what the body uses to build muscle but they're also what the body uses to create those mitochondria (energy factories) and keep them operating at full capacity. They're also what the body uses to create hormones and neurotransmitters – like the ones that help us wake up in the morning and the ones that help us rest.

The *worst* thing you can do for your health and energy levels is to maintain a diet purely made up of processed carbs. Things like chocolate bars, crisps, pies, sausage rolls – these have had all the goodness removed and all that is left is a sudden 'hit' of sugar. That causes the sugar spike and trough we talked about but it also fills you up without providing your body with everything it needs.

Honestly – packing your diet with nutrients is essentially like taking all the best bodybuilding supplements in a way that's cheaper and more effective. It boosts brain power too! Don't spend tons of money on multivitamins and supplements – just try to get a balanced, mixed diet.

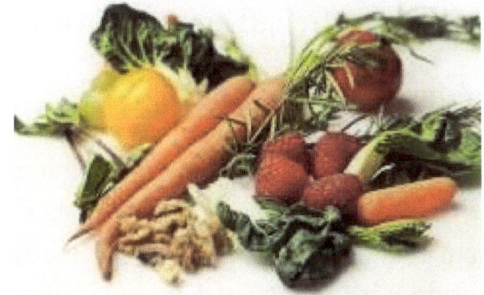

To demonstrate the importance of nutrients, here are some examples of the things that nutrients do for...

•Magnesium and zinc increase testosterone production

•CoQ10 increases mitochondrial function (found in organ meats and beef)

•Creatine helps you run further and train longer by recycling ATP (found in beef)

•Choline increases brain activity (found in eggs)

•Saturated fat is used to create testosterone (found in milk, eggs)

•Vitamin C boosts your mood (via serotonin) strengthens the immune system

•Omega 3 fatty acid (found in fish) increases cell membrane permeability – improves communication between cells

•Vitamin B12 is used to manufacture neurotransmitters

•Iron increases the ability to get oxygen around the body

•Calcium strengthens muscle contractions

•The list goes on and on...

But don't spend ages worrying about all this. Your body evolved to thrive off of a balanced and rich diet. If you just eat lots of stuff you know is healthy, you will supply your body with plenty of powerful agents to improve your brain power, strength and more.

Just eating more salad, more fruit smoothies and more meats will help you to perform better in the long term and the short term. You'll sleep better, feel healthier and enjoy more energy throughout the day.

Now Run With This Information ...

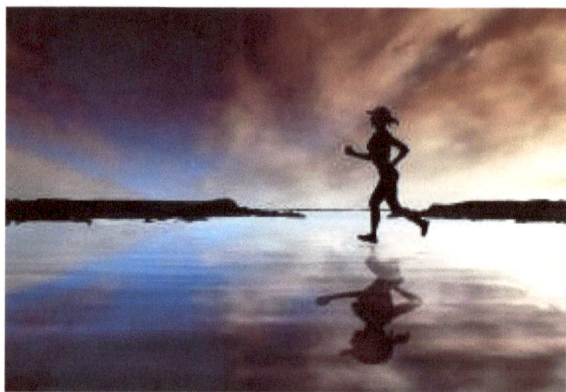

Hopefully this book has helped to convince you of the importance of energy and maintaining and managing it throughout the day. On top of that though, you hopefully now have a more complete picture of precisely what dictates your energy levels and how that impacts on your ability to work, to train and to enjoy life in your down time.

It comes down to management, planning and being smart about your routine. But it's also a matter of understanding the biology that dictates the way you feel and how you can subtly influence that to get the best from yourself.

But now comes the hard part – adapting that information to help it fit your own life and your own routine. It's worth it though: get this right and you'll be far more productive at work, far happier at home and MUCH healthier.

Cheat Sheet

Now you better understand the ebbs and flows of energy throughout your body, you should be ready to start managing it throughout the day and ensuring you always have enough energy to do the things that *you* want to do, when you want to do them.

We've gone through the theory, now it's time for practice! This cheat sheet lays out everything you need to do, remember and consider, and will help you go from tired and lethargic, to firing on all cylinders.

Recognize: Energy is Finite

We started in the book by discussing something you need to recognize when it comes to your energy: it is finite. That means you don't need to only think about time management. Just because you have time to do something, that doesn't mean that you can or *will* do it. What's equally important is your energy and if you come home from work completely drained, that means you're not going to be able to work out or to start writing a novel!

Manage Your Energy

So how do you get more energy to do the things you need or want to do?

Simple: you cut out things that sap energy from your routine.

This includes:

- Commuting – Can you do a car share? Or perhaps go into work an hour earlier or an hour later so that you skip rush hour?

- Cooking – Can you get a food delivery on a regular basis? This will help you to spend less time in the kitchen. Make sure it's a healthy one!

- Washing Up – Get a dishwasher and machine-washable pots and pans.

- Cleaning – Invest in a cleaner. Likewise, consider a robotic vacuum cleaner.

- Shopping – Set up a standing order.

- Calls – Learn to multitask. If you spend a lot of time making calls, do it when you would have been busy otherwise.

- Decisions – Decision fatigue is real. Combat it by spending less time on decisions that really don't matter – like what to wear.

- Travel – While commuting might be necessary, you can cut down other types of travel by finding a nearer gym (making a home one), by working from home some days, by finding a more local shop or by buying things in bulk.

If this doesn't free up enough energy for you, then you might have to consider cutting out something. This might mean spending less time with friends, or it might mean quitting a class after work.

If you want to add something in, something has to go!

Sleep Better

The biggest way to boost your energy levels is to sleep better. This will help you to quickly enhance your energy levels as well as to improve your overall health.

To start sleeping better, there are numerous things you can do.

A good starting point, is to go to bed earlier and try to maintain a consistent routine for going to bed and waking up. The body works based on rhythms and recognizing this is an excellent way to ensure you're able to operate on full steam when you need to.

Another tip is to regulate your temperature. Have a warm bath and then keep the room slightly cool when you're sleeping. Use the right cognitive script to help yourself feel calm and try to avoid lights and screens just before bed!

Diet

Diet is one of the key things that will improve your energy levels. The minute you start eating a more nutritious diet, you will begin to provide yourself with more of the neurotransmitters you need to stay awake, more of the protein you need to maintain your tissue, more of the vitamins and minerals that protect and enhance your immune system... etc.

The good news is that it is super easy to add some extra energy to your diet by just getting a smoothie in there once a day – or even a multivitamin and mineral tablet.

Also important is to avoid 'empty calories' and particularly processed, simple carbs. Sausage rolls, crisps, chocolates, chips... these have no place in your diet except as an occasional treat.

For starters, these foods spike your blood sugar and precede an immediate crash. Then there's the fact that they don't offer *any* useful nutrients.

Consume complex carbs and healthy fats that will provide a steady flow of energy throughout the day.

Exercise

Now you need to introduce exercise to your routine. This will boost the performance of your mitochondria, your circulation and plenty more to do with energy levels.

The key is to start an exercise regime you're likely to be able to stick to. Don't be too ambitious if you're already struggling with low energy!

And think about the easy ways you can fit exercise into your routine by reducing travel to a gym or by working out *before* your shower (so that your workout doesn't mean you have to have an extra shower every day!).

A great way to train is to use a simple circuit of a few exercises. In the book, we discuss the QUICK routine, which uses:

- Pull-Ups

- Push-Ups

- Squats/Tuck Jumps

This is enough to train the entire body and you can perform it in a quick sequence with a minute break in between each one. It will only take ten minutes, will work the entire body and will burn fat and improve your fitness in the process!

Give Yourself an Energy Boost!

There are plenty of things you can do to give yourself a quick energy boost when you need one:

- Move around

- Splash cold water on your face

- Go outside in the sun and get some vitamin D

- Listen to some music

- Eat a good energy source like a banana

- Stand in a 'power position' to release some testosterone

- Prime your mood by watching an action scene or something else that works you up

- Put yourself in a richer and more interesting environment

- Remind yourself why what you're doing matters

Now you have all the tools, all the knowledge and all the steps. Time to supercharge your energy levels!

Resource Sheet

If you want to boost your energy levels, there are a number of different methods you can use. One of the most effective is to supplement your diet with the right nutrients, nootropics and other powerful ingredients.

This resource sheet is here to help you do exactly that and to provide you with a breakdown of the best supplements for boosting your energy levels and brain power too.

Omega 3 Fatty Acid

Omega 3 fatty acid works by increasing your 'cell membrane permeability'. This essentially means that you are making the cell walls in your brain and body easier to pass through, which in turn means that electrical signals, nutrients and more can all enter the cell body (soma) for use. The result is that signals can end up bouncing through your brain at a faster rate, making you feel more awake and more alert.

Most of us get too much omega 6 and not enough omega 3. By supplementing with omega 3 and cutting out the omega 6 sources that come from things like ready meals, you should feel 5x better.

Creatine

Creatine is a supplement that is used by athletes. Its job is to convert used ATP (AMP and ADP) back into useable ATP. In doing this, you are able to get more use out of the energy that's in your body for a couple of seconds of extra endurance.

It may not sound like much but if you're lifting weights or trying to focus on a hard problem, you'll find it makes a big difference.

Vitamin D

Vitamin D is produced by the body when we get sunlight. Unlike other vitamins and nutrients, vitamin D is in many ways closer to a hormone and actually acts like a kind of 'master key' for your other hormones. Specifically, it can improve your sleep and increase testosterone, resulting in a lot more energy and much better performance.

MCT Oil

MCT oil is a type of oil that comes from coconut oil. It stands for 'medium chain triglyceride' and it's basically a unique type of fat that gets taken straight to the liver and there stimulates the production of ketones. Ketones are a useful 'alternate' source of energy that the body can use in the place of glucose. The brain actually prefers ketones for certain activities and thus you will feel more alert and awake almost instantly after consuming a little MCT.

Caffeine

Caffeine is an interesting choice for increasing your energy levels and waking up. It works by blocking the effects of adenosine, which is a neuroinhibitor and by-product of the energy process. Adenosine is what makes us feel tired at the end of the day, so caffeine can reverse this. This is perfect for when you need to get just a little more productivity out of yourself before you can switch off, but seeing as caffeine is addictive and can blunt your creativity, it's very important that you try not to become dependent on it. Use it only when needed.

Mind Map

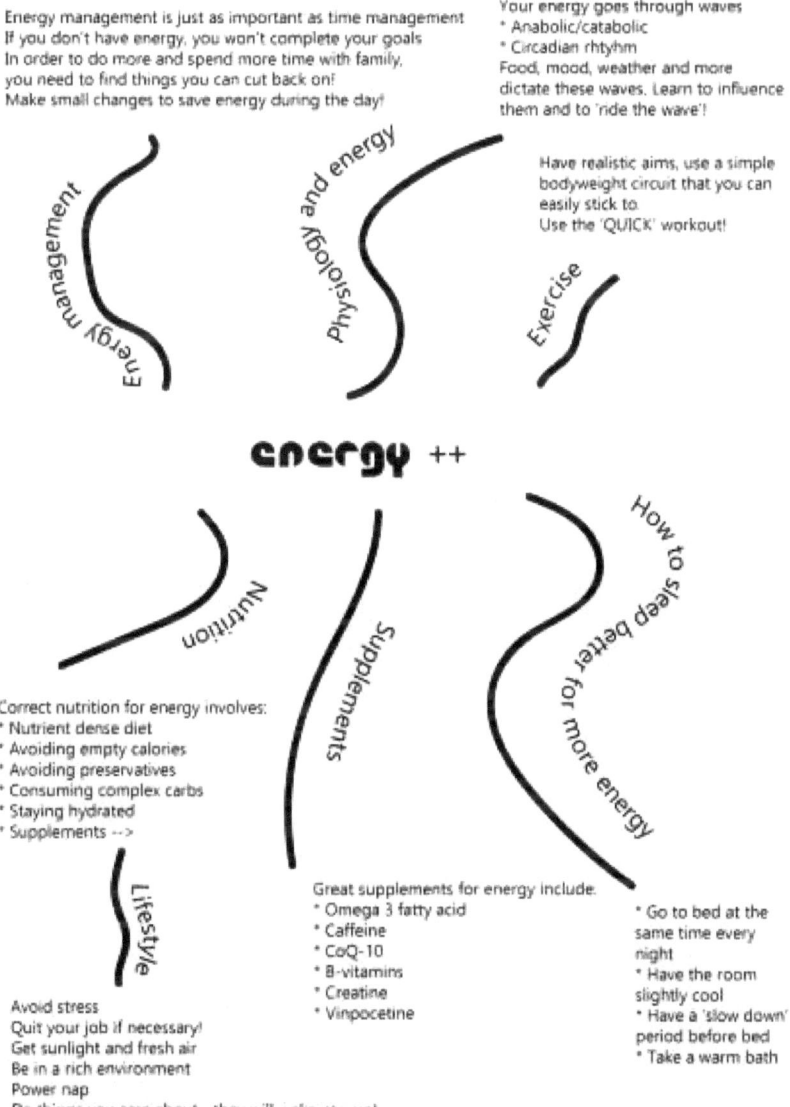

Energy management is just as important as time management
If you don't have energy, you won't complete your goals
In order to do more and spend more time with family,
you need to find things you can cut back on!
Make small changes to save energy during the day!

Your energy goes through waves
* Anabolic/catabolic
* Circadian rhtyhm
Food, mood, weather and more
dictate these waves. Learn to influence
them and to 'ride the wave'!

Have realistic aims, use a simple
bodyweight circuit that you can
easily stick to.
Use the 'QUICK' workout!

Energy management

Physiology and energy

Exercise

energy ++

Nutrition

Supplements

How to sleep better for more energy

Correct nutrition for energy involves:
* Nutrient dense diet
* Avoiding empty calories
* Avoiding preservatives
* Consuming complex carbs
* Staying hydrated
* Supplements -->

Lifestyle

Avoid stress
Quit your job if necessary!
Get sunlight and fresh air
Be in a rich environment
Power nap
Do things you care about - they will wake you up!

Great supplements for energy include:
* Omega 3 fatty acid
* Caffeine
* CoQ-10
* B-vitamins
* Creatine
* Vinpocetine

* Go to bed at the
same time every
night
* Have the room
slightly cool
* Have a 'slow down'
period before bed
* Take a warm bath

Other Relevant Books by This Author

If you would like to read more relevant books about this topic, here is a list of the Createspace links, titles and descriptions from this author:

https://www.createspace.com/6853248

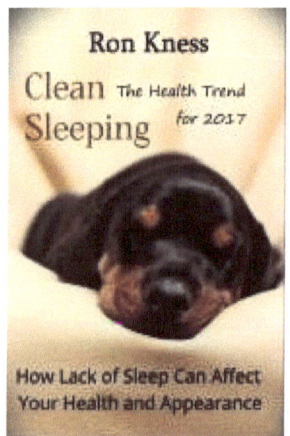

Clean Sleeping - The Health Trend for 2017: How Lack of Sleep Can Affect Your Health and Appearance

We want to be more energetic the next day . We also want to be more productive . And we want to get more sleep and of a better quality!

We can achieve ALL of these goals with the newest release from Ron Kness called *Clean Sleeping - The Health Trend For 2017*. Based on these exciting teachings, you will learn about all the dramatic benefits of restful sleep and eating foods that help people sleep better.

This book is built around a very clear, concept: feel well rested.

It's not just about ways to get the maximum amount of restorative sleep. Having great sleeping habits is linked to eating healthy. This is because some foods are more conducive to sleeping well than others

In this book, we look at all of the ways you can improve your own sleeping habits, starting with calming the mind. This book will also look at the many other steps that can be taken to support this goal, from doing meditation before retiring for the night to taking a warm bath scented with an essential oil and listening to soft music. Even the choices you make about healthy eating and creating sleep-inducing bedroom environment can have an impact on your sleeping habits.

In *Clean Sleeping - The Health Trend For 2017*, we'll cover all the bases, giving you everything you need to know to get the maximum amount of quality sleep each night. It is the most important thing you can do for your overall physical and mental health.

The good news is that getting a good night's rest is totally doable ... we show you how!

https://www.createspace.com/6845571

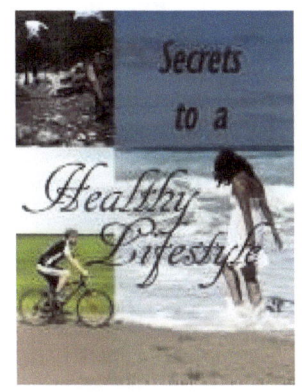

Secrets to a Healthy Lifestyle: 7 Lifestyle Changes To Make This Year the Best Yet

Along with a New Year comes the opportunity to let go of the past and start fresh and anew. It's a perfect time to get serious about getting healthy.

Don't think of it as a new year's resolution. Think of it as a brand-new start on your life. Out with the old, and in with the new. What's more is that it's not as difficult as you think. You can have less stress with a few simple daily actions, eat better by adding in more healthy food and get healthier by exercising more without feeling like it's so much work.

In addition, just a few money and time management, and unhealthy habit changes will make all the difference in your life. Finally, you'll have more time for more fun without spending tons of money. You're going to feel so much better with just a few specific changes, that you'll have the very best year you've ever had.

Turn off electronics, head for a walk in the park, have a picnic, then go grocery shopping leisurely. Make fun a priority in your life and you'll naturally be healthier, happier and have an amazing year, every year.

https://www.createspace.com/6313333

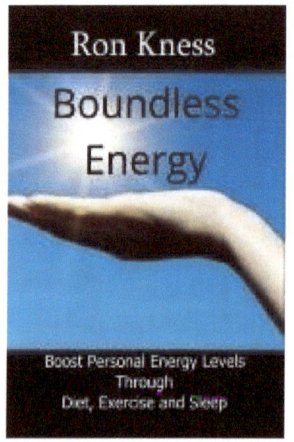

Boundless Energy: Discover How to Boost Energy Levels So You Can Get More Done, Feel Less Stressed and Live Life to the Max

Everyone is always talking about time management. There just aren't enough hours in the day for many of us and so the belief goes that if we could squeeze a little more productivity out of our time, we'd be able to accomplish our dreams, earn more money, stay more organized and enjoy more time off.

It all sounds great, except for one thing: the entire endeavor is completely misguided. Sounds harsh but in fact it's also completely true. Your problem is not with time.

You have plenty of time. If you didn't have plenty of time, you probably wouldn't have been able to watch that entire boxset of Criminal Minds Season 10 would you? And you likely wouldn't have spent so long on YouTube...

The problem isn't time – it's energy. Your energy, just like your time, is finite. Only it actually exists in somewhat smaller quantities meaning that it's all too easy to run out and end up completely exhausted. And that's when we start to use our time poorly and not get much done.

Think about it: imagine if you could jump out of bed feeling energetic first thing in the morning. What would you do with that extra hour of productivity? Hit the gym maybe?

Make some calls? Do last night's washing up so that you could live in a house that wouldn't always be untidy?

Remember when you were a little kid and you could just run around all day without ever seeming to get tired? Wouldn't it be incredible if you could get that back?

That's what we'll be looking at in this book…
• How to assess your own energy levels
• How mitochondrial function contributes to your energy levels and how to get back the mitochondrial function you had in your youth
• How to use supplements to give yourself a 'competitive edge' when it comes to energy
• How to choose superfoods that supercharge your energy
• How to avoid foods that drain your energy and slow your body down
• What type of training you can use to increase your energy
• The role of stress in energy management
• The secrets to a perfect night's sleep and how this leads to enhanced energy
• How habits and morning schedule contribute to your energy
• How more energy makes you perform better – and even be smarter!

About the Author

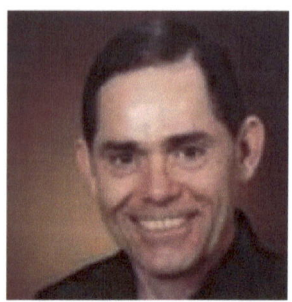

I have published over 125 books on Amazon for Kindle, CreateSpace and other publishing platforms.

While most of my books are on health and fitness in general, as I age (now 65) at the time of this writing) my topics of interest are geared toward aging baby boomers and older.

Besides my own writing, I also ghostwrite ebooks, books, reports, articles, blogs and do Kindle conversions for clients on a variety of topics.

Today my wife and I are retired from our careers and live in Gold Canyon, AZ. I now write as a retirement business where you'll find me happily sitting in my office typing away on my laptop as I work on my next book or ghostwriting project . . . that is if we are not traveling on a cruise ship - our new-found mode of travel.